Table of Contents

INTRODUCTION 4

What Is Pancreatitis? 5

What Are Symptoms of Acute Pancreatitis 8

What Are the Symptoms of Chronic Pancreatitis 10

What are the risk factors for pancreatitis? 11

What Are the Causes of Pancreatitis 12

When Should I Contact a Doctor If I Think I May Have
Pancreatitis 14

Which Types of Doctors Treat Pancreatitis 15

How Is Pancreatitis Diagnosed 16

Is There a Specific Diet for Pancreatitis 19

What Is the Medical Treatment for Acute Pancreatitis? 21

Can Pancreatitis Be Prevented 24

What Is the Outlook for a Person Who Has Pancreatitis 26

Diet for acute and chronic pancreatitis 28

Therapeutic dietary food. 31

Stage of fading exacerbation of pancreatitis........................ 34

Chronic pancreatitis in remission 36

Diet in pancreatitis, taking place in chronic form 38

Pancreatic Liquid Diet.. 50

Clear Pancreatic Liquid Diet 50

Full Pancreatic Liquid Diet... 52

Pancreatitis Diet Recipes 53

   The Modified Vegan 54

   Pancreatitis recipes 56

      Oil Free Salad Dressings................................... 56

      Chicken Vegetable Soup That Is Simply Delicious!........... 61

      Split Pea Soup Is Pancreas Friendly 64

      LOW Fat Hot Cocoa (chocolate) 71

      Vegetable Broth Recipe 75

INTRODUCTION

The term "Pancreatitis" refers to inflammation and swelling of the pancreas. The pancreas is a gland situated behind the stomach and next to the large intestine. The functions of the pancreas include releasing of digestive enzymes into the small intestine and releasing of hormones insulin and glucagon in to the blood stream. Pancreatitis or inflammation of the pancreas occurs when the powerful digestive enzymes are activated before they are released into the small intestine and they begin attacking the pancreas.

Nutrition is a vitally important part of treatment for patients with pancreatitis. The primary goals of nutritional management for chronic pancreatitis are:

- Prevent malnutrition and nutritional deficiencies
- Maintain normal blood sugar levels (avoid both hypoglycemia and hyperglycemia)

- Prevent or optimally manage diabetes, kidney problems, and other conditions associated with chronic pancreatitis
- Avoid causing an acute episode of pancreatitis

To best achieve those goals, it is important for pancreatitis patients to eat high protein, nutrient-dense diets that include fruits, vegetables, whole grains, low fat dairy, and other lean protein sources. Abstinence from alcohol and greasy or fried foods is important in helping to prevent malnutrition and pain.

Nutritional assessments and dietary modifications are made on an individual basis because each patient's condition is unique and requires an individualized plan. This Pancreatitis human diet book offers nutritional and gastrointestinal support for those with pancreatitis.

What Is Pancreatitis?

The pancreas is a gland located in the upper part of the abdomen. It produces two main types of substances:

digestive juices and digestive hormones. Inflammation of the pancreas is termed pancreatitis and its inflammation has various causes. Once the gland becomes inflamed, the condition can progress to swelling of the gland and surrounding blood vessels, bleeding, infection, and damage to the gland. There, digestive juices become trapped and start "digesting" the pancreas itself. If this damage persists, the gland may not be able to carry out normal functions. Pancreatitis may be acute (new, short-term) or chronic (ongoing, long-term). Either type can be very severe, even life-threatening. Either type can have serious complications.

Acute pancreatitis usually begins soon after the damage to the pancreas begins. Attacks are typically very mild, but about 20% of them are very severe. An attack lasts for a short time and usually resolves completely as the pancreas returns to its normal state. Some people have only one attack, whereas other people have more than one attack, but the pancreas always returns to its normal state unless necrotizing pancreatitis develops and becomes life-threatening.

Chronic pancreatitis begins as acute pancreatitis. If the pancreas becomes scarred during the attack of acute pancreatitis, it cannot return to its normal state. The damage to the gland continues, worsening over time.

The reported annual incidence of acute pancreatitis has ranged from 4.9 to 80 cases per 100,000 people. About 80,000 cases of acute pancreatitis occur in the United States each year. Pancreatitis can occur in people of all ages, although it is very rare in children. Pancreatitis occurs in men and women, although chronic pancreatitis is more common in men than in women.

What Are Symptoms of Acute Pancreatitis

The most common symptom of acute pancreatitis or pancreas pain is abdominal pain. Almost everybody with acute pancreatitis experiences abdominal pain.

The pain may come on suddenly or build up gradually. If the pain begins suddenly, it is typically very severe. If the pain builds up gradually, it starts out mild but may become severe. The pain is usually centered in the upper middle or upper left part of the belly (abdomen). The pain is often described as if it radiates from the front of the abdomen through to the back.

The pain often begins or worsens after eating.

The pain typically lasts a few days.

The pain may feel worse when a person lies flat on his or her back.

People with acute pancreatitis usually feel very sick. Besides pain, people may have other symptoms and signs.

Nausea (Some people do vomit, but vomiting does not relieve the symptoms.)

Fever, chills, or both

Swollen abdomen which is tender to the touch

Rapid heartbeat (A rapid heartbeat may be due to the pain and fever, dehydration from vomiting and not eating, or it may be a compensation mechanism if a person is bleeding internally.)

In very severe cases with infection or bleeding, a person may become dehydrated and have low blood pressure, in addition to the following symptoms:

Weakness or feeling tired (fatigue)

Feeling lightheaded or faint

Lethargy

Irritability

Confusion or difficulty concentrating

Headache

Cullen's sign (bluish skin around the belly button)

Grey-Turner sign (reddish-brown skin discoloration along the flanks)

Erythematous skin nodules

If the blood pressure becomes extremely low, the organs of the body do not get enough blood to carry out their normal functions. This very dangerous condition is called circulatory shock and is referred to simply as shock.

Severe acute pancreatitis is a medical emergency.

What Are the Symptoms of Chronic Pancreatitis

Pain is less common in chronic pancreatitis than in acute pancreatitis. Some people have pain, but many people do not experience abdominal pain. For those people who do have pain, the pain is usually constant and may be disabling; however, the pain often goes away as the condition worsens. This lack of pain is a bad sign because it probably means that the pancreas has stopped working. Other symptoms of chronic pancreatitis are related to long-term complications, such as the following:

- Inability to produce insulin (diabetes)
- Inability to digest food (weight loss and nutritional deficiencies)
- Bleeding (low blood count, or anemia)
- Liver problems (jaundice)

What are the risk factors for pancreatitis?

The major risk factors for pancreatitis are excessive alcohol intake and gallstones. Although the definition for excessive alcohol intake can vary from person-to-person, most health-care professionals suggest that moderate consumption is no more than two alcoholic beverages a day for men and one a day for women and the elderly. However, people with pancreatitis secondary to alcohol intake are usually advised to avoid all alcohol intake.

Other risk factors include

- a family history of pancreatitis,
- high levels of fat (triglycerides) in the blood,
- cigarette smoking,
- certain inherited disorders such as cystic fibrosis, and
- taking certain medicines (for example estrogen therapy, diuretics, and tetracycline).

What Are the Causes of Pancreatitis

Alcohol abuse and gallstones are the two main causes of pancreatitis, accounting for 80% to 90% of all individuals diagnosed with pancreatitis. Pancreatitis from alcohol use usually occurs in individuals who have been long-term alcohol drinkers for at least five to seven years.

Most cases of chronic pancreatitis are due to alcohol abuse. Pancreatitis is often already chronic by the first time the person seeks medical attention (usually for severe pain).

Gallstones form from a buildup of material within the gallbladder, another organ in the abdomen (please see previous illustration). A gallstone can block the pancreatic duct, trapping digestive juices inside the pancreas. Pancreatitis due to gallstones tends to occur most often in women older than 50 years of age. The remaining 10% to 20% of cases of pancreatitis have various causes, including the following:

- medications,
- exposure to certain chemicals,
- injury (trauma), as might happen in a car accident or bad fall leading to abdominal trauma,
- hereditary disease,
- surgery and certain medical procedures,
- infections such as mumps (not common),

- abnormalities of the pancreas or intestine, or
- high fat levels in the blood.
- In about 15% of cases of acute pancreatitis and 40% of cases of chronic pancreatitis, the cause is never known.

When Should I Contact a Doctor If I Think I May Have Pancreatitis

In most cases, the pain and nausea associated with pancreatitis are severe enough that a person seeks medical attention from a health-care professional. Any of the following symptoms warrant immediate medical attention:

- Inability to take medication or to drink and eat because of nausea or vomiting
- Severe pain not relieved by nonprescription medications
- Unexplained pain
- Difficulty breathing

- Pain accompanied by fever or chills, persistent vomiting, feeling faint, weakness, or fatigue
- Pain accompanied by presence of other medical conditions, including pregnancy
- The health-care professional may tell the person to go to a hospital emergency department. If a person is unable to reach a health-care professional, or if a person's symptoms worsen after having being examined by a health-care professional, an immediate visit to an emergency department is necessary.

Which Types of Doctors Treat Pancreatitis

The types of doctors that usually treat pancreatitis are emergency medicine doctors, primary care physicians, internal medicine specialists, hospitalists, critical-care specialists and occasionally gastroenterologists and/or surgeons, depending upon the severity of the disease.

How Is Pancreatitis Diagnosed

When a health-care professional identifies symptoms suggestive of pancreatitis, specific questions are asked about the person's symptoms, lifestyle and habits, and medical and surgical history. The answers to these questions and the results of the physical examination allow the health-care professional to rule out some conditions and make the correct diagnosis. In most cases, laboratory tests are needed. The tests check the functioning of several body systems, including the following:

- Pancreas, liver, and kidney functions (including levels of pancreatic enzymes amylase and lipase)
- Signs of infections, for example, fever or fatigue
- Blood cell counts indicating signs of anemia
- Pregnancy test
- Blood sugar, electrolyte levels (an imbalance suggests dehydration) and calcium level

- Results of the blood tests may be inconclusive if the pancreas is still making digestive enzymes and insulin.
- Diagnostic imaging tests are usually needed to look for complications of pancreatitis, including gallstones.

Diagnostic imaging tests may include the following:

X-ray films may be ordered to look for complications of pancreatitis as well as for other causes of discomfort. This may include a chest X-ray.

A CT scan is like an X-ray film, only much more detailed. A CT scan shows the pancreas and possible complications of pancreatitis in better detail than an X-ray film. A CT scan highlights inflammation or destruction of the pancreas. Occasionally an MRI is ordered.

Ultrasound is a very good imaging test to examine the gallbladder and the ducts connecting the gallbladder, liver, and pancreas with the small intestine.

Ultrasound is very good at depicting abnormalities in the biliary system, including gallstones and signs of inflammation or infection.

Ultrasound uses painless sound waves to create images of organs. Ultrasound is performed by gliding a small handheld device over the abdomen. The ultrasound emits sound waves that "bounce" off the organs and are processed by a computer to create an image. This technique is the same one that is used to look at a fetus in a pregnant woman.

Endoscopic retrograde cholangiopancreatography (ERCP) is an imaging test that uses an endoscope (a thin, flexible tube with a tiny camera on the end) to view the pancreas and surrounding structures.

ERCP is usually used only in cases of chronic pancreatitis or in the presence of gallstones.

To perform an ERCP, a person is first sedated. After sedation, an endoscope is passed through the mouth, to the stomach, and into the small intestine. The device then injects a temporary dye into the ducts connecting the liver, gallbladder, and pancreas with the small intestine (biliary ducts). The dye makes is easier for the health-care professional to see any stones or signs of organ damage. In some cases, a stone can be removed during this test.

Is There a Specific Diet for Pancreatitis

The diet for people with acute pancreatitis consists of bowel rest for a few days. Bowel rest means no food or liquid intake by mouth. Consequently, patients need to be provided fluids and nutrition intravenously in the hospital while the pancreas is given time to recover. The patient is then slowly advanced to oral intake starting off with clear fluids and then soups.

Patients with chronic pancreatitis are suggested to have a low-fat diet (maximum 20 g/day), high carbohydrates in are advised to eat small sized and more frequent meals (about 5 to 6 per day). If the pancreas develops a flare, the patient should go back to bowel rest for about a day or so but not to become dehydrated by taking oral fluids. If symptoms don't resolve, medical care should be sought immediately. Patients with either chronic or acute pancreatitis strongly advised not to drink any alcoholic beverages.

Are There Home Remedies That Soothe or Cure Pancreatitis

For most people, self-care alone is not enough to treat pancreatitis. People may be able to make themselves more comfortable during an attack, but they will most likely continue to have attacks until treatment is received for the underlying cause of the symptoms. If symptoms are mild, people might try the following preventive measures:

Stop all alcohol consumption.

Adopt a liquid diet consisting of foods such as broth, gelatin, and soups. These simple foods may allow the inflammation process to get better.

Over-the-counter pain medications may also help. Avoid pain medications that can affect the liver such as acetaminophen (Tylenol and others). In individuals with pancreatitis due to alcohol use, the liver is usually also affected by the alcohol.

What Is the Medical Treatment for Acute Pancreatitis?

In acute pancreatitis, the choice of treatment is based on the severity of the attack. If no complications are present, care usually focuses on relieving symptoms and supporting body functions so that the pancreas can recover. Most people who are having an attack of acute pancreatitis are admitted to the hospital.

Those people who are having trouble breathing are given oxygen.

An IV (intravenous) line is started, usually in the arm. The IV line is used to give medications and fluids. The fluids replace water lost from vomiting or from the inability to take in fluids, helping the person to feel better.

If needed, medications for pain and nausea are prescribed.

Antibiotics are given if the health-care professional suspects an infection may be present.

No food or liquid should be taken by mouth for a few days. This is called bowel rest. By refraining from food or liquid intake, the intestinal tract and pancreas are given a chance to start healing.

Some people may need a nasogastric (NG) tube. The thin, flexible plastic tube is inserted through the nose and down into the stomach to suck out the stomach juices. This suction of the stomach juices rests the intestine further, helping the pancreas recover.

If the attack lasts longer than a few days, nutritional supplements are administered through an IV line.

What Is the Medical Treatment for Chronic Pancreatitis

In chronic pancreatitis, treatment focuses on relieving pain and avoiding further aggravation to the pancreas. Another focus is to maximize a person's ability to eat and digest food.

Unless people have severe complications or a very severe episode, they probably do not have to stay in the hospital.

Medication is prescribed for severe pain.

A high carbohydrate, low fat diet; and eating smaller more frequent meals help prevent aggravating the pancreas. If a person has trouble with this diet, pancreatic enzymes in pill form may be given to help digest the food.

People diagnosed with chronic pancreatitis are strongly advised to stop drinking alcohol.

If the pancreas does not produce sufficient insulin, the body needs to regulate its blood sugar, and insulin injections may be necessary.

What about Surgery for Pancreatitis

If the pancreatitis is caused by gallstones, an operation to have the gallbladder and gallstones removed (cholecystectomy) is likely. If certain complications (for example, enlargement or severe injury of the pancreas, bleeding, pseudocysts, or abscess) develop, surgery may be needed to drain, repair, or remove the affected tissues.

Can Pancreatitis Be Prevented

The following recommendations may help to prevent further attacks or to keep them mild: Completely eliminate alcohol because it is the only way to reduce the chance of further attacks in cases of pancreatitis caused by alcohol use, to prevent the pancreatitis from worsening, and to prevent the development of complications that can be very serious or even fatal.

Eat small frequent meals. If in the process of having an attack, avoid solid foods for several days to give the pancreas a chance to recover.

Eat a balanced diet high in carbohydrates and low in fats because may help individuals decrease the risk for pancreatitis since it is likely these actions will decrease the risk for gallstones, a major risk factor for pancreatitis.

If pancreatitis is due to chemical exposure or medications, the source of the exposure will need to be found and stopped, and the medication will need to be discontinued.

Don't smoke

Maintain a healthy weight

Exercise regularly

What Is the Outlook for a Person Who Has Pancreatitis

Most people with acute pancreatitis recover completely from their illness unless they develop necrotizing pancreatitis. The pancreas returns to normal with no long-term effects. Pancreatitis may return, however, if the underlying cause is not eliminated. Some 5%-10% of people develop life-threatening pancreatitis and may be left with any of these chronic illnesses, or even die due to complications of pancreatitis:

Kidney failure

Breathing difficulties

Diabetes

Brain damage

Chronic pancreatitis does not resolve completely between attacks. Although the symptoms may be similar to those of acute pancreatitis, chronic pancreatitis is a much more serious condition because damage to the pancreas is an ongoing process. This ongoing damage can have any of the following complications:

Bleeding in or around the pancreas: Ongoing inflammation and damage to the blood vessels surrounding the pancreas can lead to bleeding. Fast bleeding can be a life-threatening condition. Slow bleeding usually leads to low red blood cell count (anemia).

Infection: Ongoing inflammation makes the tissue vulnerable to infection. The infection can form an abscess that is very difficult to treat without surgery.

Pseudocysts: Small fluid-filled sacs can form in the pancreas as a result of ongoing damage. These sacs can become infected or rupture into the lower abdominal cavity (peritoneum), causing a serious infection called peritonitis.

Breathing problems: The chemical changes in the body can affect the lungs. The effect is to reduce the amount of oxygen the lungs can absorb from the air a person breathes. The level of oxygen in the blood drops to lower than normal (hypoxia).

Pancreas failure: The pancreas may become so severely damaged that it is unable to carry out its normal functions. Digestion of food and regulation of blood sugar - both very important functions - are affected. Diabetes and weight loss often result.

Pancreatic cancer: Chronic pancreatitis can encourage the growth of abnormal cells in the pancreas, which can become cancer. The prognosis for pancreatic cancer is very poor.

Diet for acute and chronic pancreatitis

Diet in pancreatitis, especially when chronic, to observe is very important. You should eat as much protein as possible and you need to reduce or completely eliminate fats and carbohydrates, especially sugar, which consists of carbohydrates on 99%, exclude fried foods and any products containing coarse fiber. It is advisable to start taking vitamins. There should be little, but often, that is, 5-6 times a day.

Pancreas is necessary to ensure normal functioning of the body: it is due to the digestive juice that it secrete in the lumen of the duodenum that the basic components of food products – proteins, fats and carbohydrates – are split. As a result of the digestion process occurring on this part of the digestive tract, simpler compounds are obtained, which enter the general bloodstream after absorption of the intestinal mucosa. Thus, nutrients, amino acids and vitamins necessary for the flow of metabolic processes in cells and for the construction of tissues, are formed from foods in the area of the duodenum and reach all organs and systems of the body.

In addition, the pancreas produces insulin, necessary for the normal course of carbohydrate metabolism, and lipokine, which prevents fatty degeneration of the liver.

The cause of pancreatitis is most often the abuse of fatty foods and alcoholic beverages. The disease can occur in both acute and chronic forms. Diet in pancreatitis depends on the features of the course of the pathological process: an acute period requires a more strict relationship to the diet and foods eaten.

In acute or chronic inflammation of the pancreas, cardinal digestive disorders occur, including:

changes the pH of the medium of the small intestine to the acidic side, as a consequence of this the patient feels heartburn, burning in the intestine;

enzymes accumulate inside the gland, begin the process of self-digestion of tissues, causing severe pain in the abdominal region in the navel region, on the right;

toxic substances accumulate, self-poisoning of the organism takes place;

impaired insulin secretion, provokes sugar diabetes.

The pathogenesis of pancreatitis develops according to the type of acute or chronic inflammation. The principle of treatment of all forms of pancreatitis includes, according to indications:

drug substitution therapy, taking into account the nature of the inflammation, the patient's condition;

Therapeutic dietary food.

Proper nutrition at the stages of rehabilitation of pancreatitis, especially after discharge from the hospital significantly increases the chances of complete recovery or stabilization of pathology.

It is in the home, often violated the principle of dietary nutrition. Meanwhile, it is important to follow the immutable rules of the medical diet. Especially since diets do not contain expensive products, cooking them is the simplest, including: grinding, boiling, steaming.

During an exacerbation of an attack of a pancreatitis, before arrival of an ambulance, it is supposed to apply cold compresses on a site of a pain, usually a pain with a substrate. During this period, it is allowed to drink mineral water (for example, Borjomi, Narzan). The daily volume of liquid to five or six glasses, with normal urination. Simple liquids suppress the release of pancreatic juice into the lumen of the duodenum, reduce the pain syndrome, and remove toxins from the body.

When a person falls ill in a medical institution, the patient will be assigned a dietary diet, developed by a dietitian.

Sets of products, names of diets, other information are approved by the order of the Ministry of Health of the Russian Federation No. 330 from 5 August 2003 г "About measures for the improvement of therapeutic nutrition in medical institutions of the Russian Federation" and the letter of the Ministry of Health of the Russian Federation from 07.04.2004 No. 2510 / 2877-04-32. These documents are valid at the time of writing.

For an illustration of principles of diets at a pancreatitis we have made extracts from the specified documents. Numbered diets, officially, in medical institutions are not used. With pancreatitis, diets with an abbreviation SHCHD and VBD are recommended.

In acute pancreatitis in the first two days the patient is prescribed a hunger. It is allowed to drink only a broth of dog rose or mineral water – one glass up to five times a day. On the third day, it is allowed to eat, but only low-calorie foods, excluding fats, salt and meals, which increase the secretion of gastric juice and stimulate the process of gassing in the intestine. All the following days, while the patient is in the hospital, he must strictly adhere to the diet indicated by the doctor!

Stage of fading exacerbation of pancreatitis

Recommended diet, taking into account the mechanical and biochemical sparing of the intestinal mucosa. This food includes:

physiological level of the main components of food – proteins, lipids, carbohydrates;

increased amount of fat and water-soluble vitamins;

a low content of substances that irritate the intestinal mucous membranes, including food seasonings;

It is forbidden to use spicy, salty, spicy, smoked.

Ways of cooking: steaming. Food is ground, wiped, small pieces of ready-made food are allowed. The temperature of food served on the table should not exceed 65 0 C. The recommended amount of meals is five to six per day.

The maintenance in a daily portion of the general protein 90 grams, animal origin 40 grams.

Containing in the daily portion of fats, 80 grams, vegetable 30 grams.

Carbohydrate content in a daily portion of 300 grams, easily assimilated 60 grams.

Energy value of 2480 kilocalories.

After the symptoms of acute pancreatitis subsided, it is better to switch to soups, use lean meats and fish, fresh cottage cheese, cereals and vegetables, as well as puddings. Products such as fruit juices, honey, jam, sugar – should be reduced or excluded from the diet. Before going to bed are useful laxative drinks: yogurt, yogurt, etc. It is important to completely abandon fatty foods, muffins, fried fish, fat, sour cream, salted and smoked dishes, marinades, onions, garlic, radishes, alcoholic beverages.

Recommended diet for pancreatitis in acute form should be observed from six months to a year. Practically one hundred percent the health of the patient depends on how strictly he adheres to the prescription of the doctor regarding the diet. It is important to remember that all errors in the diet are immediately reflected in the status of the pancreas.

Chronic pancreatitis in remission

In this version, a different approach to feeding the patient. During this period, nutritionists recommend to include in the diet an increased protein content, the physiological rate of fat. More complex approach to carbohydrates. Diet at the stage of remission involves:

protein is allowed slightly above the physiological norm;

the norm for fats and complex carbohydrates in the form of cereals;

below the norm include in the diet of sugar, honey, jam, cakes, sweet buns, also below normal cooking salt.

In this version, it is prohibited to eat irritating mucous membranes of the gastrointestinal tract. These products include vinegar, alcohol, other substances used as seasonings.

Dishes are prepared boiled, stewed, baked, steamed. It is allowed to serve food in a wipe, not wiped. Feeding at short intervals, in small portions 4-6 once a day. Food is served in a warm form. Its temperature is not more than sixty degrees Celsius.

The maintenance in a daily portion of the total protein 120 grams, including animal origin 50 grams.

The maintenance in a daily portion of fats 90 grams, vegetable fats 30 grams.

The maintenance in a daily portion of carbohydrates 350 grams, easily assimilated 40 grams.

Energy value of 2690 kilocalories.

Diet in pancreatitis, taking place in chronic form

Chronic pancreatic pancreatitis develops in most cases against the background of an acute disease. At the same time, it can be primary if the patient suffers from liver cirrhosis, hepatitis, duodenal pathology, cholelithiasis, allergies, atherosclerosis, alcohol abuse.

The diet with pancreatitis, which takes place in chronic form, is considered the main one in the treatment of this disease. In the remission phase, the number of calories contained in the daily diet should correspond to the physical load. It is recommended to take food up to six times a day, not forgetting about food, which is characterized by a laxative effect.

It is important to monitor the daily intake of protein. Since it is necessary for the normal course of recovery processes, it must be consumed in sufficient quantities – up to 130 grams per day, with only 30% protein should be plant origin.

In the diet of a patient suffering from chronic pancreatitis, it is necessary to include beef, veal, rabbit meat, chicken, turkey, low-fat pork. Prohibited: lamb, fat pork, as well as goose meat, ducks and game. If the patient is worried about frequent pain, meat dishes are cooked in chopped form or cooked for a couple, you can not bake dishes in the oven, fry and stew. Similarly, low-fat fish is prepared.

Meat and fish dishes with a low fat content help the patient avoid fatty liver degeneration, which is of great importance in chronic pancreatitis. A similar property is also found in homemade cottage cheese, but only if it is non-acidic and fresh, store cottage cheese is not recommended.

Milk in its pure form with chronic pancreatitis is often poorly tolerated, so it is better to add it to cereals, soups, jelly when cooking them. Even if the milk is tolerated well by the patients, they should not be abused, drinking only half a glass of warm milk per day in small sips. It is much more useful for people suffering from pancreatitis, fresh sour-milk products. Forbidden for exacerbation of the disease, cheese in the remission phase can be eaten in small amounts provided that you feel well. Cheese should be low-fat and not sharp. Whole eggs are excluded from the diet, at the same time, protein omelettes are cooked for steaming, meals with whipped proteins, in addition, eggs can be present as an additive in other dishes.

Proteins of vegetable origin can be represented by rice, yesterday's bread, breadcrumbs, semolina, oatmeal, buckwheat, pasta. Bean cultures should not be eaten with pancreatitis.

Fats in the diet should be no more than 70 grams, and 80% of them are animal fats, they should be eaten together with other dishes and food. It is better to put the oil in a ready dish just before eating, vegetable oil is acceptable only if it is well tolerated. Culinary fats, margarine, beef and pork fat are prohibited.

Carbohydrates in the daily diet should contain no more than 350 grams, they can be represented by sugar, honey, jam, syrup. From products rich in carbohydrates, biscuits, semolina, oatmeal, buckwheat, pearl barley, rice, pasta are allowed. Also, patients are allowed to eat potatoes, carrots, beetroot, pumpkin, zucchini, squash. Vegetable dishes should be cooked on steam or on water, you can eat vegetable steam pudding. Boiled vegetables should be eaten in a grated form with the addition of cereal broth.

Of fruits, non-acid varieties of apples are recommended: ripe fruits can be baked, wiped, cooked from them, compote, and a compote of dried fruits is also useful.

Of all the sauces, the best is considered a béchamel based on milk and flour, and the flour is not passaged, and the salt is added very little.

First course (soups from cereals, vegetables, can be on milk, meat from low-fat varieties of meat, fish, as well as sweet soups from fruit).

Main dishes (boiled beef meat, poultry, fish, omelet from chicken eggs).

Products containing cereals (porridge, pasta, white bread, black, vegetable oil).

Dairy, sour-milk products (milk 2,5%, dairy products, butter).

Berries, fruits, vegetables (ripe, sweet) in a raw, baked form, carrots, beets – boiled, like dressing soups, as side dishes and independent dishes.

Dessert (digestible carbohydrates in pancreatitis are limited, that is below the physiological norm, jam, honey, sugar).

Beverages (tea with milk, vegetable, fruit juices).

Specialized Products (a mixture of protein composite dry) Add fat and water-soluble vitamins.

It is also important not to overeat, cutting the daily amount of food to 2,5 kilograms, taking into account the drunk liquid. Food is often and in small portions.

Following all the rules of nutrition in pancreatitis can significantly improve the effectiveness of therapy in general.

The number of products must be calculated on the basis of the above normative documents.

Here is an approximate daily diet menu for pancreatitis:

The first meal (7: 00- 7: 30): boiled beef, oatmeal in milk, tea.

The second meal (9: 00-9: 30) omelet, baked apple, broth of wild rose.

The third meal (12: 00-13: 00): vegetable soup, beef soufflé, pasta, jelly from sweet berries, compote.

The fourth meal (16: 00-16: 30): cottage cheese and tea.

The fifth meal (20: 00-20: 30): souffle fish, tea.

As you can see, in a diet with pancreatic pancreatitis, all dishes are made from lean meat and fish – and then only in a boiled option. Fried foods are prohibited. You can eat dairy products with a minimum percentage of fat. From the liquid it is desirable to drink only natural juices and compotes and tea.

All kinds of alcohol, sweet (grape juice) and carbonated drinks, cocoa, coffee

Products of animal origin: offal, including the first category, meat and lard pork, fatty fish, all smoked products, spicy, fried, fast food based on extractives.

Vegetable products: legumes, mushrooms, spinach, sorrel, onions, bakery products based on buttery dough.

Desserts: chocolate, fatty creams.

Figs, grapes, bananas, dates.

Confectionery, chocolate, ice cream, jam.

Salo, cooking fats.

Hard boiled eggs, whole egg dishes, fried eggs

Is Goat Milk Permitted? This is a fairly fatty product, which is difficult to perceive pancreas. It is twice as fat as a cow. Peoples whose diet from time immemorial includes goat's milk are more adapted to the product. In unaccustomed organism milk can provoke upset stomach. The product should be included in the diet gradually, starting with small portions. If the body responds well (there is no nausea and vomiting, a normal stool), portions can be increased.

Is the matzoni allowed? This sour-milk product is allowed in pancreatitis. Before eating, you need to pay attention to the fat content of the milk from which it is made. Milk of high fat content is not recommended for use.

Are muffins, puff pastry, cakes allowed? At the stage of exacerbation, the listed products can not be. At the stage of remission, yeast baking is allowed in small amounts. The menu can include items made from puff pastry. As for gingerbread, the quality and quantity of glaze is important (if there are insulin disturbances, they should be minimally sweet). Inexpensive products are covered with a glaze made on palm or coconut oil, which is extremely harmful to the gland.

Is cinnamon allowed? Cinnamon is a seasoning, which can be bought in a specialized store or which is supplied by distributors. What is presented in hypermarkets in a packetized form is an inexpensive option, called cashier. With such an "analogue" are related myths about its health-improving effect in type 2 diabetes. This is not the work of the gland, but the response of insulin receptors in the tissues. There are no official confirmations to that. With regard to this cinnamon, it increases the production of digestive juice, which is undesirable in the event of an exacerbation of the disease. (See also: Benefits and harm of cinnamon)

Are offal products allowed? The heart, stomach and liver are not contraindications for pancreatitis, provided that the right preparation is made. Such products can be eaten in boiled or stewed form. Fried eating them is not recommended.

Is processed cheese, bread, chocolate, coffee allowed? Cream cheese should be the easiest, that is, without any seasonings and additives. Bread can be included in the menu. Chocolate is allowed in small quantities. Coffee is not recommended at any stage of the disease. As an option – you can drink coffee with milk and in small quantities.

Is rice, olive oil allowed? Rice is allowed. Olive oil can be filled with salads and other dishes.

Is brine allowed? At the stage of remission, a small amount of brine does not harm, but it should not be drunk in large amounts.

Is salted bacon allowed? Salo is hard for the liver and gall bladder. When it is used, the pancreas suffers again. Outside the stage of exacerbation, fat is allowed, however in small amounts (up to two slices a day up to two times a week).

Pancreatitis is an inflammation of the pancreas. The cause of pancreatitis is overlapping the duct gland stones from the gallbladder, a tumor or cyst. In such a situation, the outflow of digestive juices with enzymes into the small intestine fails. These pancreatic enzymes accumulate with.

In the acute form of the disease, the pains are localized under the spoon in the upper part, the left and right hypochondrium, if the entire gland is affected, the pains have a shingling character. Also, the patient develops vomiting with an admixture of bile, which does not bring him relief.

Cryphaea is the most effective remedy for the treatment of pancreatitis, ulcerative formations and other diseases of the digestive system. This is due to the plant's unique curative substance s-methylmethionine. Its properties consist in the ability to normalize the acid balance of the gastrointestinal.

There is a mass of medicinal plants that have a beneficial effect on the functional state of the pancreas and contribute to the improvement of its activity. Herbal medicine should be considered as an additional tool in complex medication. Most often, the treatment is done in a hospital. The sick person is prescribed pain medication, and a special system is developed to eliminate inflammation. When pancreatitis in the stomach sometimes accumulate air and liquid, which can cause attacks of severe vomiting. If there are such symptoms in the treatment.

Survived on a dropper of glucose. On the ninth day, forcibly pushed food scar scar forty. Appetite appeared on 15 day. Very fond of delicacies. Gusses, ducks, salami European, smoked meat, beer, dry wine. Neither of which is now impossible. Melon and watermelon (not mixing) you can eat only in the remission stage, in moderation!

Pancreatic Liquid Diet

After the pancreas has cooled down and the pain faded then the next step will probably be to use a pancreatic liquid diet to slowly reintroduce you to food. The diet that you will be prescribed are usually called a clear liquids diet and a full liquids diet. The idea that Doctors use is that food needs to be introduced slowly to allow the pancreas to slowly start full functioning again.

Clear Pancreatic Liquid Diet

Clear liquids will generally be introduced first then if the pancreatitis tolerates this well either a full liquid diet or a solid diet will be prescribed. Clear Liquids are described as those that can be seen through. These liquids are more easily absorbed by the intestines and cause less stress to the pancreas.

Even though they contain some nutrition they are incapable of meeting the bodies energy requirements for more than a couple of days. This type of diet would include things like:

Bouillon soup without vegetables or noodles.

Coffee.

Fruit juices without pulp.

Gelatin

Popsicles

Soft drinks

Sports drinks

Tea

Water

After several days or more recovering from an attack of Pancreatitis it's amazing how good even gelatin can taste. It's almost like your taste buds have been reset and are tasting the food you are eating anew.

Full Pancreatic Liquid Diet

In some cases after you tolerate a pancreatic clear liquid diet instead of allowing a person to start a solid diet Doctors will want to have you try a full liquid diet. These pancreatic liquid diets include everything in a clear liquid diet but also include:

Cream of wheat

Fruit juices with pulp

Honey

Jelly

Milk, milkshakes and ice cream

Nutrition supplement drinks like Ensure or Boost

Pureed meats or vegetables

Soups with only a few solids

Vegetable juices

Yogurt and pudding

Pancreatitis Diet Recipes

pancreaitis diet recipes is a brand new category and my hope is that you'll find it to be helpful in your journey to better health.

Most pancreatitis diet recipes you can find on the internet are not safe. They are conjured up by those who really don't know what can be eaten in relative safety and what foods should never be eaten.

When coming out of an acute attack I've heard of people being fed or told they can eat some of the most dangerous foods, by hospital employees (doctors, nutritionists, etc). Those who suffer from chronic disease have no real guidance. They have no guidance because, let's face the truth, you are worth more sick than welf you're well you don't visit the hospital ER rooms. You don't need routine office visits. You don't need prescription drugs or surgical procedures.

It is absolutely amazing to me how little the medical profession knows or is willing to tell about what is safe and what isn't safe for pancreatitis patient to eat. This holds true for nutritionists as well. As a result ... Safe pancreatitis diet recipes are extremely hard to find.

This new book category will endeavor to bring you a variety of decent tasting foods you will be able to enjoy in relative safety. Remember ... If you are still experiencing symptoms because you have not healed it is best to eat what I have termed as a modified vegan meal plan.

The Modified Vegan

Modified vegan simply means your food comes from plant sources, not animal sources. True vegans do not eat animal products however ... They do eat foods that you and I should not. Just because something grows in the ground or on a bush or tree which grows in the ground doesn't mean it is safe. If you haven't read my post on pancreatitis diet basics you should do that. You should also read all the other posts about diet.

Vegans eat high fat foods such as nuts and seeds. Nuts and seeds are not safe. They eat and use oils in cooking. Oils are not safe. They eat avocado, coconut, soybeans and soy products which are not safe. Not for those of us who suffer with pancreatitis.

Once you have healed enough to be symptom free you can then begin to explore the short list of relatively safe animal foods. Now ... IF you have had only one mild attack and there isn't a lot of damage or an underlying cause that hasn't been addressed (be advised a pancreas doesn't simply wake up one morning and decide to become inflamed) you have an extremely good chance of healing totally, never having to worry about chronic disease but...

IF you are suffering from chronic pancreatitis or you have had more than one or two acute pancreatitis attacks and have not yet been diagnosed with chronic pancreatitis (even though you have ongoing, unrelenting symptoms) I would highly suggest the first place to start should be to begin a food diary.

You will quickly note that this section is a little premature if you really want to learn what you should and should NOT eat. Rather than take my word for it doing a proper food diary is the ONLY way you can learn what foods work for you and what foods do not work for you. Then ... This section containing pancreatitis diet recipes will become a valuable resource

Pancreatitis recipes

Oil Free Salad Dressings
Oil free salad dressings can be a tasty treat for those who need to avoid oil consumption. The following salad dressings are oil free and perfect for people like us (pancreatitis patients). Salads are great for those who have pancreatitis.

Salads (greens and other veggies) are safe food. Salads are full of vegetables (leafy greens, cruciferous, tubers, legumes, etc) which contain tons of essential nutrients, minerals and antioxidants (phytonutrients).

The problem with salads is that they taste somewhat bland to awful without something to dress them up and add that taste bud anticipation. And that is where good oil free salad dressings shine.

You'll need a clear shaker cup. If you don't have a clear one any kind of shaker cup will do. You could even mix the ingredients with a spoon, cup or small bowl if you don't have a shaker cup. Whatever works!

Once you have your dressing made you can either drizzle dressing onto your salad or you can dump the dressing on the salad (in a bowl) and toss it till it's all mixed. Whatever works for you.

The following dressings are my favorites but you can vary any of them in any way you choose. It is your taste pallet that counts! So use my ideas to create variations of your own.

Honey Mustard

This is the basic dressing. You can create variations of your own besides the two that follow. Add or detract ingredients depending upon your own taste. You'll need:

Apple cider vinegar (3 tablespoons)

Honey mustard (3 tablespoons)

Shake together and drizzle or dump and toss. This dressing goes well on all kinds of greens or greens with legumes. It also tastes great on chicken and fish!

Honey Sweet Hot Mustard

You will need:

Apple cider vinegar (6 tablespoons)

Sweet hot mustard (3 tablespoons)

Honey mustard (3 tablespoons)

Shake ingredients together and either drizzle on your salad or dump and toss. This dressing goes well on all kinds of greens or greens with legumes. It also tastes great on chicken and fish!

Balsamic Honey Mustard

You'll need these ingredients:

Apple cider vinegar (3 tablespoons)

Balsamic vinegar (3 table spoons)

Honey mustard (6 tablespoons)

Shake ingredients together and drizzle over your salad or dump it and toss. Enjoy!

Honey, Lime Juice & Mint

This oil free salad dressing is designed for a nice fruit salad. Choose any kind of fruit (especially berries) and poor or drizle this dressing on and enjoy an eating extravaganza!

You'll need:

1/2 cup of wild honey

1 lime

Fresh organic mint

Squeeze the lime into the 1/2 cup of wild honey, add some mint (about a 1/2 teaspoon) and mix. Then drizzle or dump and toss. You can increase the amount of dressing to fit your needs.

Lime Juice & Ketchup

This one is super easy too! All you need is:

8 limes

2 tables spoons of ketchup

Just shake this concoction in a shaker, drizzle or poor over and toss a salad made of cucumber, tomato, celery, onion (and anything else you want like legumes, fish, shrimp etc) and you have a tasty salad! You can use this dressing to make Ceviche!

Chicken Vegetable Soup That Is Simply Delicious!

I created a chicken vegetable soup that was so lip smacking good that I just have to share it. It should be completely safe because it is made with nothing that is unsafe for those of us who suffer with chronic pancreatitis. The picture is NOT my soup. I am one of the very few people on the planet that does not have a cell phone with a camera or a camera I could use to take digital pictures. So I apologize but I'm serious ...

This chicken vegetable soup is so good you may never make any other kind of chicken vegetable soup. The broth is delightfully sweet (not over sweet, just a hint of sweetness), the soup itself boasts a filling four servings of chicken breast pieces (skinless chicken breasts) and large chunks of vegetables. It will satisfy even the heartiest man sized appetites and is full of protein, vitamins and minerals.

You can create any variations you wish using this recipe for chicken vegetable soup however; adding or subtracting ingredients will obviously change the flavor of the soup so give this specific recipe a try before you create variations. You'll like it.

One of the things you need to remember about me is that I do NOT measure. I am a dumper or a do-it-to-my-taste kinda guy. So I'll list the ingredients with approximate amounts as a starting point and you'll have to go from there. In other words you have to taste it while cooking to see if you need to add more of anything. Naturally I'm being conservative with the spices because once in you can't take them out but you can always add more to your particular taste.

What you'll need:

1.A large pot (5 quarts) with cover

2. 4 Yukon Gold potatoes

3. 6 good sized carrots

4. 3 large parsnips

5. 5 celery stocks

6. Celery leaves (about half a cup)

7. One large yellow onion

8. Salt (1/2 teaspoon)

9. Pepper (1/2 teaspoon)

10. Bay leaves (2 or 3)

11. Basil (1/2 teaspoon)

12. Parsley (1 teaspoon)

13. Garlic (4 – 6 fresh crushed or 1 teaspoon of garlic powder)

14. Thyme (1/4 teaspoon)

Cut up two fresh, skinless chicken breasts (more if you like) and add the chunks to about 3 cups of water (it looked like about 3 cups, maybe it was 4 lol). My pot was about half full of water before I added the chicken. Bring to a boil on high heat and once boiling back down the heat until you have a gentle boil. Cover the pot and cook the chicken for 30 minutes.

While the chicken is cooking wash, peel and cut your vegetables into nice, good sized chunks. And at the 30 minute cooking mark add ALL the vegetables and spices then cook for another 30 minutes or until the vegetables are to your liking for tenderness. Make sure you taste the soup and see if it is to your liking as far as spices. If it needs more ofsome spice add to taste. Once you have the soup broth to your taste liking set the soup aside to "rest" for 10 minutes and then dig in!

Split Pea Soup Is Pancreas Friendly

Split pea soup is one of my favorite soups. I can eat it any time of year in fact I just made a batch so I could write this recipe. Remember I usually "dump" and never measure so it is hard for me to say exactly how I make foods.

But in order to share with you what I eat in order to keep my pancreas from being unhappy I am starting to write down recipes for foods like split pea soup. By the way ... Split pea soup is a wonderful rst solid food to eat after coming out of an acute pancreatitis attack or with symptomatic chronic pancreatitis (after the fast and juice phase) and starting out on what are usually safe solid foods again.

One of the benets of split pea soup is the protein content. According to the package of the peas I use there is 11 grams of protein in a 1/4 cup of split peas.

Green peas are extremely low in fat and a mega source of vitamin K, manganese, ber, B1, copper, folate, phosphorus and vitamin C. Peas also contain a unique assortment phytonutrients that can lower inammation (yep like in the pancreas) and the risk of cancer,

According to this site I use to check out food nutrition there is 16 grams of protein per cooked cup plus a ton of other nutrients. When I look up split pea soup on the same site I nd that there is 10 grams of protein per cup of soup. So I gure my soup is going to boast about the same protein and nutrition content.

Most soup recipes (including pea soup) you'll read about in cookbooks, online or on can and box labels will include oil of some kind. Of course for those who have recurring acute pancreatitis (do to an underlying condition), chronic pancreatitis or sphincter of oddi dysfunction oil (pure fat) is not a good thing.

In order to avoid oil and other high fat ingredients often included in food recipes we, as pancreatitis patients, need to improvise, adapt, overcome. That is often easier said than done and I have found the best way is to simply cook at home, writing, or making up your own recipes.

Let's Make Split Pea Soup!

First we are going to make my basic split pea soup. Underneath the basic version I'll give you other ingredients you can add in order to make variations.

Note that making the variations will often change the avor to something more atuned to a vegetable soup with a split pea base.

Ingredients you'll need:

1 pound bag of split peas

1 quart Swanson's Organic Vegetable Broth NOTE: If you are a celiac like me you may not want to use this broth because it contains wheat!

Supposedly the wheat has been processed in some manner to conform to FDA "gluten free" standards. I choose to make my own vegetable broth which is a pain but necessary for my health.

2 nice big onions (chopped or diced)

2 – 3 green onions (chop them all with the green tops)

2 yukon gold potatoes (chopped or diced)

3 medium carrots (diced)

3 stalks of celery with leaves (chopped)

4 cloves of garlic (pressed) or 1 tsp of garlic powder (add more if you like)

1/4 tsp thyme

2 nice bay leaves

1 tsp of black pepper

1 tsp salt (or to taste)

1 tbsp of dried parsley

Directions:

1. Empty the pound of split peas into a 5 quart pan. Put them under the faucet (running almost hot water) and rinse the peas thoroughly swishing the peas with your hand. Pour o water (will be a soapy looking water) being careful not to pour out the peas. Repeat until the water runs clear.

2. Once the water is clear and the peas are clean ll the pan with water until there is about one inch of water above the peas. Set it on the stove (high heat) and bring to a boil. Once peas come to a boil, stir them and make sure none are sticking to the bottom of the pan, then decrease heat to medium and continue to slowly boil the peas for about an hour or until they begin to turn into soup. Do NOT add

ANYTHING until the peas are breaking down. Just peas and water. You might have to add some water so keep your eye on the peas you do not want them to burn!

3. Once the peas have begun to break down add the potatoes, the carrots, the celery, the onions and simmer for another 15 minutes. Stir up nicely. Watch the peas, don't let them burn.

4. Add the vegetable broth and spices and then simmer for another 15 minutes. Stir the soup and check to see if it looks like soup.

5. Check the peas and veggies for tenderness.

6. When the soup looks like this in the pan it is ready to serve

7. Dish your soup up and cover the top in green onion!

8. EAT!

Variations: Making variations to the above soup is simple. Just add extra vegetable ingredients. You can add:

1. Corn (frozen or fresh) which supplies more protein and other nutrients

2. Green peas (frozen or fresh) for more protein, a sweeter taste and more nutrients

3. Spinach (frozen or fresh) for more protein and tons of killer nutrients

4. Green beans (frozen or fresh) for a distinctive green bean avor and nutrition

5. Lima beans (frozen) for more protein and nutrition

You can add one of the above, several or all. Adding other vegetables (you can add almost anything) does change the avor.

Each new vegetable adds

it's own taste and nutrition. Experiment. Have fun and enjoy eating safe split pea soup.

LOW Fat Hot Cocoa (chocolate)

How would you like a nice cup of LOW Fat Hot Cocoa? You know, hot chocolate!

When the chill is in the air something chocolate, cooking on the stove can smell, well, delicious and ... On winter evenings there is nothing like a good cup of hot chocolate!

For those who have pancratitis, can tolerate no fat milk and love chocolate this is a way to get that chocolate x you crave.

Pancreas Friendly LOW Fat Hot Cocoa (chocolate)

Before you try making low fat hot cocoa I'd suggest making sure your pancreas tolerates no fat milk. Some people do, some people don't. I can tolerate some every now and then but denitely not every day. So test no fat milk rst then try this low fat hot chocolate!

Here's how to make homemade hot choclate that actually tastes pretty darn good and has very little fat!

Ingredients you need:

1/2 cup sugar

1/4 cup HERSHEY'S Cocoa (2 grams of fat)

3/4 teaspoon ALCOHOL FREE vanilla extract

4 cups (1 qt.) NO FAT milk

1/3 cup hot water

Marshmallows (if desired)

Directions

1. Stir together sugar, cocoa and salt in medium saucepan; stir in water. Cook over medium heat, stirring constantly, until mixture comes to a boil. Boil and stir 2 minutes. Add milk; stirring constantly, heat to serving temperature. Do Not Boil.

2. Remove from heat; add vanilla. Beat with rotary beater or whisk until foamy. Serve topped with marshmallows, if desired. Five 8-oz. servings.

Dark Chocolate Variation:

RICH, Dark LOW Fat Hot Cocoa (chocolate)

Same as above but add an additional 2Tbsp of Hershey's Special Dark

Cocoa (1 gram of fat)

Whether you tolerate no fat milk or not you'll have to nd out if you want a cup of hot chocolate. As you'll note this makes about a quart of hot chocolate (about 5 cups) so each cup has LESS than 1 gram of fat as far as I can gure.

If you only drink one cup (suggested) save the rest in the pan, put it in the fridge and re-warm it later or drink it as chocolate milk lol

Good luck, hope it works and you like it!

More Variations:

SPICED COCOA: ADD 1/8 teaspoon ground cinnamon and 1/8 teaspoon

ground nutmeg. Serve with cinnamon stick, if desired.

SWISS MOCHA: ADD 2 to 2-1/2 teaspoons powdered instant coee.

CANADIAN COCOA: ADD 1 – 2 teaspoons of pure maple syrup.

MICROWAVE SINGLE SERVING: Combine 1 heaping teaspoon HERSHEY'S

Cocoa, 2 heaping teaspoons sugar and dash salt in microwave-safe cup or mug. Add 2 teaspoons cold milk; stir until smooth. Fill cup with milk.

Microwave at HIGH (100%) 1 to 1-1/2 minutes or until hot. Stir to blend; serve.

Vegetable Broth Recipe

I'm going to give you another of my secret weapons. A food for pancreatitis that I still use to this day, my special pancreatitis vegetable broth. This broth can be used anytime. It is especially good for those just coming out of an acute pancreatitis attack or if you are still suffering pain and nausea from chronic pancreatitis.

I know that I have recommended fresh organic vegetable juice or low sodium V8 juice. The fresh organic vegetable juice made from tomato, carrot, spinach, broccoli, celery, onion and garlic is hard to beat and is much better than this broth but ...

What do you do if you don't have a juicer?

You either buy a juicer so you can juice organic vegetables or you buy low sodium V8 juice.

Unfortunately the V8 juice has been processed so much there is very little nutrient value. V8 juice is rich in potassium but lacks in everything else.

Pancreatitis Vegetable Broth Recipe

This is not a fancy recipe and I'm not a chef so don't expect a miraculous, mouth-watering delicacy. It's just a vegetable broth that your inamed pancreas should easily tolerate and will be far superior in nutrients than V8 juice. Be sure to use ORGANIC vegetables for your pancreatitis vegetable broth.

2 tomatoes

2 potatoes

2 carrots

1 cup of sliced celery

1 cup of chopped broccoli

1 cup of scrunched up spinach leaves

1/2 cup of sliced onion

1 clove of fresh garlic (smashed)

Salt and pepper to taste

Make sure everything was washed good before preparation. Cut the stem out of the tomatoes, put them in a pot and then crush them. Next peel the potatoes, set the potatoes aside and put the skins in a pot . Peel the carrots and put the skins in the pot and save the carrots with the potatoes.

Put them into a bowl that will be large enough to hold all the vegetables you are putting into the pot (you remove the potato and carrot skins later and keep the rest).

Throw all the other ingredients into the pot and add enough water to cover the vegetables. If you want a bigger pot of broth just use more vegetables. Turn heat up and watch for the water to steam. NOT BOIL just steam.

Check the temp with a gauge. You want it at 180/190. Just under boiling.

Cover the pot and simmer at that temp for about 10 minutes to kill any bugs (E coli, norovirus, salmonella). Then turn the heat o and let the vegetable broth steep for another 5 – 10 minutes. This leaches the vitamins and minerals from the potato and carrot skins and the other veggies.

Now get a strainer and strain the broth so you have nothing but a nice vegetable broth. Viola you have my pancreatitis vegetable broth. Salt and pepper to taste and drink up.

You can also use it to make vegetable soups etc. Just remember the more you cook stu the less nutrient value it retains because heat kills live enzymes, vitamins, antioxidants, phytonutrients and a lot of minerals. Remove the skins and keep the other veggies. You can now freeze the leftover veggies, including the peeled potatoes and carrots and use them to make soup or boiled taters, carrots and onions. Nothing but the skins go to waste unless you don't like soup or potatoes, carrots and onions.

Give my pancreatitis vegetable broth a try and see how it works for you.

Made in the USA
Monee, IL
12 March 2021

62575025R00046